5 MINUTES SOMATIC EXERCISES FOR WEIGHT LOSS

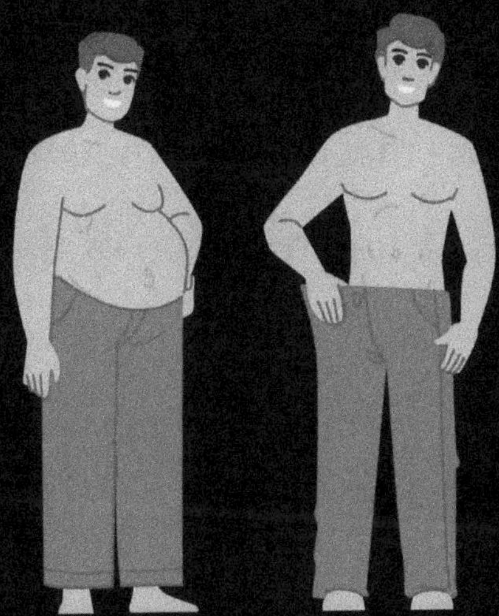

Quick and Easy Workouts with 4 Weeks Program to Burn Calories and Have your Desired Body Weight

Dr. Diane Reyes

Table of Contents

Introduction

It was the first day of spring, and Jeff felt a glimmer of motivation as he peered down at the scale. The numbers hadn't budged all winter long, just like his workout routine and waistline. Jeff craved change, but his busy life didn't leave much time for lengthy workouts or complicated diets. "There must be an easier way," he sighed.

Like many of us, Jeff struggled to find a practical, sustainable approach to weight loss that fit within his hectic lifestyle. The thought of exhausting gym sessions or depriving himself of food until summer seemed daunting and frankly unappealing. If you share these frustrations, I have good news: meaningful change is possible in as little as 5 minutes per day.

This book will introduce you to somatic exercises - simple, accessible mind-body movements that help you lose weight by reducing stress, engaging your core, improving mindfulness, and cultivating body awareness. In just 5 minutes each day, you can spark lasting improvements through brief but powerful somatic sequences. No fancy equipment or harsh diets required!

Too often, we force unrealistic workout regimes on ourselves that quickly fizzle out. The somatic path respects your busy life while guiding you toward better health through microscopic changes that compound over time. If you're ready to get off the rollercoaster of short-lived diet and fitness obsessions, somatic exercises offer a refreshing, sustainable approach.

Join Jeff as he evolves his mindset around exercise and nutrition, learns to distinguish emotional eating from true hunger, and develops a nurturing inner voice to stick to this gentle routine. His journey models realistic expectations, self-compassion for missteps, and small victories that ultimately accumulate into weight loss success.

Don't waste another minute punishing yourself into exhaustion for underwhelming results. Let this book open your eyes to a calm, mindful way to shape your body that integrates seamlessly into your life. Are you ready to give yourself the gift of health in just 5 minutes each day? Let's begin...

Why Somatic Exercises?

Somatic exercises are a unique form of exercise that involve slow, mindful movements to connect the mind and body. "Soma" means the body in its wholeness, emphasizing the integration of body and mind. Somatic exercises are different from traditional exercises in that the focus is not on burning calories or building muscle. The goal is to cultivate body awareness, improve posture and alignment, release tension, and increase mind-body connection.

In today's busy world, many people struggle to find time for lengthy workouts. Somatic exercises offer a convenient way to retain the benefits of exercise even with a busy lifestyle. The slow, gentle movements can be done in as little as 5 minutes per day. The mindful approach also provides stress relief and mental focus. Let's explore the 5-minute somatic workout and all its benefits for health and wellbeing.

The 5-Minute Approach to Weight Loss

Here is a simple 5-minute somatic routine to jumpstart your weight loss efforts:

- Seated Breathwork (1 minute)
Sit comfortably with eyes closed. Inhale deeply through the nose, expanding the belly. Exhale slowly through the mouth, drawing the navel in. Repeat for 1 minute, focusing on deep belly breaths.

- Neck Stretches (1 minute)
Drop your right ear to right shoulder, feeling the stretch on the left side of neck. Inhale as you return your head to center, then exhale as you drop left ear to left shoulder. Repeat slowly with deep breaths.

- Shoulder Circles (1 minute)

Sit tall with shoulders relaxed. Circle shoulders up, back, down and forward. Reverse direction. Move slowly with control.

- Pelvic Tilts (1 minute)

Sit with knees bent, feet on floor. Tilt pelvis forward, flattening lower back, then tilt pelvis back. Move slowly, focusing on using core muscles.

- Calf Stretches (1 minute)

Stand facing wall with hands on wall for support. Step right foot back with toes pointed forward. Bend left knee, keeping right leg straight. Hold for 30 seconds, then switch legs.

This simple routine wakes up the body, aids circulation, relieves muscle tension, engages the core, and stimulates the vagus nerve to aid digestion. Over time, this encourages weight loss by reducing cortisol levels and boosting metabolism. The mind-body focus also cultivates mindfulness and self-awareness.

Benefits of Somatic Exercises

Regular somatic exercise, even for just 5 minutes daily, provides many benefits:

- Improves posture and body alignment to reduce pain and injury risk

- Releases muscle tension and allows deeper relaxation

- Enhances mind-body connection and interoception (awareness of inner body sensations)

- Boosts circulation and lymphatic flow

- Stimulates the vagus nerve which controls key functions like digestion, heart rate, and breathing

- Reduces cortisol and balances the nervous system

- Increases body awareness and proprioception

- Fosters mindfulness and focus

- Accessible to all fitness levels

The integrative approach of somatic movement allows you to address body, mind and spirit in as little as 5 minutes a day. The exercises can be done anywhere, without equipment or preparation. Start with just 5 minutes per day, focusing on mindful, full-body movement.

Over time, this can lead to reduced stress, deeper mind-body awareness, easier weight management, and greater embodiment. Try somatic exercises for an accessible daily routine to enhance your overall wellness.

Getting Started

Somatic exercises provide an accessible way to improve your health and potentially lose weight, in as little as 5 minutes per day. By setting realistic goals, creating a simple routine, and committing to consistency, you can make somatic exercises a sustainable habit.

Setting Realistic Weight Loss Goals

It's important to have realistic expectations when using somatic exercises for weight loss. Extreme weight loss goals and rapid results are unrealistic. Aim for a gradual, maintainable approach instead. Here are some sensible weight loss goals to strive for with regular somatic exercise:

- Lose 1 to 2 pounds per week. Losing at 1-2 pounds per week is a safe, sustainable rate for most people. Rapid weight loss is harder to maintain long-term.

- Reduce body measurements by 2 inches in 2 months. The number on the scale is not the only measure of progress. Losing inches around your waist, hips, and other areas indicates positive change.

- Increase strength and endurance. Improved strength and endurance from somatic exercises will make you feel better and aid your weight loss efforts.

- Make sustainable lifestyle changes. The ultimate goal is developing long-term habits, not just short-term weight loss. Somatic exercises support sustainable lifestyle changes.

- Focus on how your clothes fit. When the fit of your clothing improves from somatic exercises, that's a tangible sign of your progress.

By setting these types of realistic, holistic goals, you can maintain motivation as you slowly but surely improve your health.

Creating a 5-Minute Exercise Routine

It's easy to build a 5-minute somatic exercise routine into your day. Try this sequence:

- 1 minute seated breathwork. Deep, mindful breathing to begin connecting with your body.

- 1 minute neck and shoulder stretches. Reduce tension in common problem areas.

- 1 minute shoulder circles. Improve posture and prepare for movement.

- 1 minute pelvic tilts. Engage your core muscles.

- 1 minute calf stretches. Increase circulation and flexibility.

Perform this sequence daily, moving slowly and consciously. Breathe deeply throughout. You can also try different 5-minute somatic sequences like side bends, figure 8 hip circles, heel raises, knee rotations, and more. Experiment to prevent boredom, while keeping the routine realistic. The key is consistency in those 5 minutes each day.

Importance of Consistency

Like any lifestyle change, consistency is vital to see results with somatic exercises. Here are 3 reasons consistency matters:

1. Habit Building. It takes time for a new habit to become automatic. Maintain your 5-minute routine daily until it sticks.

2. Cumulative Effects. The changes are gradual, but performing somatic exercises consistently allows the benefits to compound.

3. Accountability. You're more likely to maintain your routine when you hold yourself accountable day after day.

Aim to perform your 5-minute somatic sequence at the same time each day. Link it with an existing habit like your morning coffee or evening meal. Track your exercises on a calendar. Find an accountability partner to check in with. Small actions performed consistently can lead to lasting change.

The mind-body integrative benefits of somatic exercises make them a worthwhile wellness habit. Start with realistic goals, customize a 5-minute routine you can maintain, and emphasise consistency in your practice. In this accessible way, somatic exercises support weight loss and improved health over time. Stick with it and you may be amazed by the changes 5 minutes can create.

Breathing Techniques

Proper breathing techniques are a vital part of somatic exercises. Conscious, controlled breathing has many benefits for both the mind and body. Let's explore three breathing techniques to enhance your somatic practice.

Deep Breathing for Relaxation

Deep belly breathing triggers the relaxation response in the body. It's a foundational breathing technique for somatic exercises.

To practice deep breathing:

- Find a comfortable seated position. Close your eyes.

- Place one hand on your belly. Breathe in slowly through your nose, feeling your belly expand.

- Exhale slowly through pursed lips, pressing out as much air as you can. Feel your belly contract.

- Repeat for 5-10 deep, slow breaths. Focus on breathing down into the belly.

- Notice how you feel calmer, grounded, and more connected to your body.

The key is breathing deeply from the diaphragm, not shallow chest breathing. Full, cleansing exhalations also help trigger relaxation.

Perform deep breathing at the start of your somatic exercises to centre yourself and relieve stress.

Diaphragmatic Breathing for Core Engagement

The diaphragm is a dome-shaped muscle located below your lungs. It contracts downward during inhalation, helping draw air into the lungs while stabilising the spine. Diaphragmatic breathing technique consciously engages this core muscle.

To practice diaphragmatic breathing:

- Lie on your back, knees bent, with one hand on your chest and one on your belly.

- Breathe in slowly through your nose, feeling your belly press into your hand. Your chest hand should remain still.

- Tighten your abdominal muscles as you exhale through pursed lips. Feel your belly hand move inward.

- Continue for 1-2 minutes, focusing on belly expansion as you inhale and contraction as you exhale.

Diaphragmatic breathing strengthens the diaphragm muscle while stimulating your abdominal muscles and vagus nerve. Use it during core-focused somatic exercises like pelvic tilts.

Breath Awareness in Daily Activities

Breath awareness is about tuning into your breathing patterns throughout your day. Notice how your breathing changes in different situations. Are you holding your breath when tense? Is your breath shallow at your computer? Somatic breathing isn't just for scheduled exercises.

Ways to build breath awareness:

- Observe your breathing before answering the phone or replying to an email. Avoid holding your breath.

- Set reminders to check your breath while working. Release any tension with deeper inhales.

- Scan your body periodically. Feel the expansion and contraction of breathing in different areas.

- Walk mindfully, coordinating steps with long, mindful inhalations and exhalations.

- Notice if emotions like stress or excitement alter your breathing. Consciously relax it.

Developing breath awareness strengthens the mind-body connection. The more you tune into your breathing patterns, the more you can regulate them for relaxation, energy, or core engagement. Make breathwork a somatic habit throughout your day.

Mindful breathing is integral to somatic exercises. Deep belly breathing triggers relaxation, diaphragmatic breathing engages your core, and breath awareness enhances mind-body control. Consciously cultivate these breathing techniques as part of your somatic practice for greater benefits. The simple act of tuning into your breath can de-stress your body, focus your mind, and deepen your inner awareness.

Mindful Eating Practices

Developing mindful eating habits is an important complement to somatic exercise for weight loss. By distinguishing emotional eating from physical hunger and cultivating awareness, you can build a healthier relationship with food.

Mindful Eating vs Emotional Eating

Mindful eating means listening to your body's actual hunger signals, whereas emotional eating is consuming food for reasons other than physical hunger. Here's how to identify mindful vs emotional eating:

Mindful eating occurs when you:

- Notice physical hunger signs like a growling stomach
- Eat slowly and attentively
- Pause halfway through a meal to check if you're still hungry
- Stop when full and content

Emotional eating occurs when you:

- Feel a sudden urge to eat without physical hunger
- Eat mindlessly or while distracted
- Keep eating past fullness
- Use food to cope with stress or boredom

Tuning into your body's signals through breath awareness and checking in with your emotions can help discern between physical and emotional hunger.

Somatic Approaches to Improve Eating Habits

Somatic exercises cultivate mind-body awareness - a skill that can support mindful eating too. Here are 3 somatic approaches to improve eating habits:

1. Breath awareness: Take a few deep belly breaths before eating to center yourself in your body. Check for actual hunger rather than just appetite.

2. Seated meditation: Practice 5 minutes of stillness and calm before eating. Observe any emotions or cravings behind the urge to eat.

3. Conscious chewing: Chew slowly, noticing flavors and textures. Pause between bites to check in on fullness levels.

The somatic state of presence helps foster new habits like eating only until 80% full,chewing thoroughly, and moderating portion sizes.

Developing a Healthy Relationship with Food

Along with mindful eating techniques, cultivating a sense of joy and gentle moderation around food is key for weight loss and somatic health:

- Food as sustenance: Shift focus to viewing food as nourishment rather than just indulgence. Apply moderation and wisdom in your food choices.

- Balancing pleasures: Allow yourself to enjoy favorite foods in moderation while emphasizing wholesome eating and portion control.

- No guilt: Avoid labelling foods as "good" or "bad" which leads to guilt. Practice detachment from food emotions.

- Self-compassion: Treat yourself kindly throughout the process. Small lapses are part of the journey.

Mindful eating means a balanced, normal relationship with food. Stay connected to your body's needs through breath awareness while also developing equanimity around food choices. The somatic path emphasises progress over perfection.

By distinguished mindful from emotional eating and cultivating moment-to-moment awareness, you can build sustainable eating habits that support weight loss and somatic wellbeing. Rather than food obsession or restriction, the goal is internal balance and lasting change. Bring a sense of peace to your eating practices through somatic exercises and mind-body connection.

Tracking Progress

Tracking your progress is an important part of any fitness routine, including somatic exercise. Using journaling, physical measurements, and celebrations of achievements can help you stay motivated on your weight loss journey.

Journaling for Awareness

Keeping a journal supports the mindfulness aspect of somatic exercises. Dedicate 5 minutes after your daily somatic session to write about:

- Energy levels - Note your mood and energy before/after exercise.

- Muscle engagement - Record which muscles you felt working.

- Breath awareness - Describe your breathing rhythm and depth.

- Mind-body awareness - Note any somatic aha moments.

- Gratitude - Express appreciation for your body's abilities.

Regular journaling allows you to tune into subtle mind-body changes. Over time, progressive somatic awareness becomes visible.

Monitoring Physical Changes

Along with subjective assessments like journaling, measure objective data to quantify somatic exercise results:

- Weight - Weigh yourself once weekly under consistent conditions. Expect an average loss of 1-2 lbs per week.

- Body measurements - Measure your waist, hips, chest, thighs, arms monthly. Even without major weight loss, reductions in inches indicate positive change.

- Body fat percentage - Use calipers or a smart scale to track fat loss over time. Improved body composition is a better metric than weight alone.

- Before/after photos - Take monthly photos wearing minimal, consistent clothing. The visual changes can be motivating.

- Fitness assessments - Record timed planks, pushups, jogs in place to benchmark strength and endurance gains.

Review your numbers regularly, but don't obsess over daily fluctuations. The data will reveal your somatic exercise results over time.

Celebrating Achievements

Don't forget to celebrate progress and non-scale victories like:

- Completing 30 straight days of somatic exercise

- Feeling your posture and alignment improve

- Advancing to longer plank holds or more reps

- Achieving a new personal record on an exercise benchmark

- Fitting into a smaller clothing size

- Receiving compliments on your physique changes

- Having more energy, less pain, better sleep

Take time to reward and congratulate yourself for both small and big accomplishments. It will help you appreciate the positive impact of your dedication and keep you motivated.

Consistent tracking provides tangible proof of your somatic exercise results. Journal mind-body insights, record physical changes, and acknowledge your hard work. Stay centered in the day-to-day practice rather than getting attached to specific outcomes. Trust that the simple act of showing up for your body will lead to progress over time. Tracking allows you to reflect on how far you've come, which fuels motivation to continue your somatic journey.

Common Challenges and Solutions

When using somatic exercises for weight loss, you may encounter some common obstacles. Understanding typical challenges and how to address them will help you stick to your routine and continue making progress.

Overcoming Plateaus

Hitting a weight loss plateau after an initial period of progress is very common. It's easy to get frustrated when the scale stops moving, but it doesn't mean your efforts aren't working. Here are 5 tips for pushing past plateaus:

1. Re-calculate your calorie needs since they change as you lose weight. Adjust your diet accordingly.

2. Increase exercise intensity with added reps, sets, or advanced moves to spur further progress.

3. Up your cardio with more frequent or longer walks, jogs, or swims.

4. Try a modified intermittent fasting approach like limiting eating to an 8-hour period each day.

5. Check for overlooked sources of extra calories like sauces, oils, snacks, or alcoholic drinks.

Stay patient and keep fine-tuning your routine. The scale will start dropping again with consistency.

Dealing with Stress and Emotional Triggers

Stress and emotions like anxiety, boredom, or depression can derail your somatic exercise efforts. Use these strategies to get back on track:

- Do a 5-minute seated somatic breathing exercise to relieve stress and re-center.

- Go for a mindful walk to decompress and refocus.

- Write in a journal to process your feelings and release negativity.

- Share your struggles with an understanding friend or in an online support group.

- Remind yourself of your "why" for doing somatic exercises and the progress you've made.

- Consult a counselor or therapist if emotions chronically overwhelm your coping skills.

Be kind to yourself on off days. Reflect on what triggered you, employ healthy stress relief tactics, and start fresh tomorrow.

Adapting Exercises for Different Fitness Levels

It's important to modify somatic exercises based on your current fitness to avoid injury or discouragement. Here are some examples:

For low fitness levels:

- Do seated instead of standing movements.

- Hold stretches for less time, and focus on gentle movements.

- Reduce number of reps, hold planks on knees instead of toes.

- Use lighter weights or resistance bands.

- Take brief breaks between exercises as needed.

For high fitness levels:

- Increase number of reps and time held for strength moves.
- Add plyometric moves like squat jumps.
- Use heavier weights or advanced bodyweight moves like single-leg planks.
- Decrease rest between sets to keep heart rate elevated.
- Add HIIT (high intensity interval training) like sprinting and jogging.

Adapt and progress your routine to match your abilities. Be patient with yourself initially but keep challenging your body over time.

Persistence and self-compassion are key when encountering obstacles with somatic exercise. Adjust your routine, cope with stress intentionally, and be flexible to get back on track toward your weight loss goals.

Core Activation Exercises

Pelvic Tilts

Starting Position:

Recline on your back with your knees bent and feet resting flat on the floor

Exercise:

Inhale and engage your pelvic floor muscles.

Exhale, gently tilt your pelvis upward, pressing your lower back into the floor.

Inhale, release the tilt, allowing a natural arch in your lower back.

Repeat this gentle rocking motion, coordinating with your breath.

Abdominal Contractions

Starting Position:

Get sitted or stand comfortably with a straight spine.

Exercise:

Inhale deeply, expanding your belly.

Exhale slowly, contracting your abdominal muscles as if you're pulling your navel toward your spine.

Hold the contraction for a moment while maintaining steady breath.

Inhale and release the contraction.

Repeat, focusing on the engagement of your abdominal muscles.

Twisting Waist Movements

Starting Position:

Stand with feet hip-width apart, arms relaxed at your sides.

Exercise:

Inhale, lengthening your spine.

Exhale, gently rotate your torso to one side, keeping your hips stable.

Inhale back to the center, maintaining good posture.

Exhale and twist to the opposite side.

Repeat, feeling the engagement in your obliques and core muscles.

Seated Russian Twists

Starting Position:

Get seated on the floor with your knees bent and feet flat.

Lean back slightly, maintaining a straight back.

Exercise:

Interlock your hands and rotate your torso towards one side.

Come back to the centre and twist in the opposite direction.

Engage your core throughout, ensuring controlled movements.

Continue this rhythmic twisting motion, syncing with your breath.

Cat-Cow Stretch

Starting Position:

Get on your hands and knees, wrists under shoulders, and knees under hips.

Exercise:

Inhale, arching your back and dropping your belly (Cow Pose).

Breath out, rounding your spine and tucking your chin to your chest (Cat Pose).

Repeat this flow, connecting breath with movement.

Focus on engaging your core as you transition between poses.

Bicycle Crunches

Starting Position:

Lie on your back, hands behind your head, and legs lifted.

Exercise:

Get one knee toward your chest while simultaneously twisting your torso to touch the opposite elbow.

Extend the bent leg while bringing the other knee towards your chest, twisting to touch the opposite elbow.

Continue this pedaling motion, engaging your core with each movement.

Plank with Hip Dips

Starting Position:

Begin in a plank position, forearms on the ground, body in a straight line.

Exercise:

Turn your hips towards one side, lowering them towards the floor.

Come back to the center and repeat the movement on the other side.

Maintain a stable plank position throughout, focusing on controlled hip movements.

Leg Raises

Starting Position:

Lie on your back, legs straight, and arms at your sides.

Exercise:

Inhale, engage your core, and lift both legs towards the ceiling.

Exhale, slowly lower your legs toward the floor without letting them touch.

Inhale, raise your legs back up, maintaining control.

Repeat, feeling the activation in your lower abdominal muscles.

Side Plank

Starting Position:

Lie on one side, elbow directly beneath your shoulder, legs stacked.

Exercise:

Raise your hips, forming a straight line from head to heels.

Hold the position, engaging your core and avoiding sagging or tilting.

Breathe deeply and maintain the side plank for the duration of the exercise.

Hollow Body Hold

Starting Position:

Recline on your back with arms stretched overhead and legs extended.

Exercise:

Lift your legs and upper body simultaneously, forming a slight 'U' shape.

Activate your core, ensuring your lower back stays pressed against the floor.

Hold the position, breathing steadily, and feeling the entire core working.

Rolling Like a Ball

Starting Position:

Sit on the floor with knees bent, feet flat, and hold onto your shins.

Exercise:

Inhale, round your spine, and lift your feet off the ground, balancing on your sit bones.

Exhale, roll back, and then inhale to roll back up to the starting position.

Focus on controlled, smooth movements, engaging your core throughout.

Standing Side Bend

Starting Position:

Stand with feet hip-width apart, arms relaxed at your sides.

Exercise:

Inhale, raise one arm overhead, and exhale, bending your torso to the opposite side.

Inhale to return to the center and switch to the other side.

Keep your core engaged and feel the stretch along your sides.

Squat with Oblique Twist

Starting Position:

Stand with feet shoulder-width apart.

Exercise:

Lower into a squat position.

As you rise, twist your torso to one side,

bringing the opposite knee towards your chest.

Return to the squat and repeat on the other side.

Engage your core for stability and balance.

Reverse Crunches

Starting Position:

Lie on your back, legs lifted towards the ceiling, and hands beneath your hips.

Exercise:

Exhale, lift your hips off the ground, bringing your legs towards your face.

Inhale, lower your legs back towards the ceiling without letting them touch the floor.

Focus on using your lower abdominal muscles for the movement.

Standing Knee-to-Elbow Crunch

Starting Position:

Stand with feet hip-width apart and hands behind your head.

Exercise:

Lift your knee towards your elbow on the same side, crunching your obliques.

Return to the starting position and switch to the other side.

Maintain a controlled pace, feeling the contraction in your core.

Mobility Exercises

Neck and Shoulder Rolls

Starting Position:

Sit or stand with a straight spine.

Exercise:

Inhale, gently roll your shoulders backward in a circular motion.

Exhale, roll your shoulders forward.

Coordinate with neck rolls, moving your head in a circular motion.

Repeat for the duration, focusing on releasing tension.

Spinal Flexibility Movements

Starting Position:

Stand with feet shoulder-width apart.

Exercise:

Breath in, arch your back, and lift your chest towards the ceiling.

Exhale, round your spine, bringing your chin towards your chest.

Repeat this flowing motion, promoting flexibility in your spine.

Hip Circles

Starting Position:

Stand with feet hip-width apart.

Exercise:

Circle your hips clockwise, emphasising the movement from your pelvis.

After a few circles, reverse the direction counterclockwise.

Focus on smooth, controlled hip movements, engaging your core.

Ankle Rolls

Starting Position:

Sit or stand with one foot lifted off the ground.

Exercise:

Rotate your ankle clockwise for several rotations.

Reverse the direction counterclockwise.

Switch to the other ankle.

Perform this exercise to enhance ankle flexibility.

Wrist and Hand Stretches

Starting Position:

Get your arms extended in front of you, palms facing down.

Exercise:

Flex and extend your wrists, moving your hands up and down.

Rotate your wrists clockwise and counterclockwise.

Stretch your fingers by gently pulling them back and holding.

Seated Forward Bend

Starting Position:

Get sitted with legs extended straight in front of you.

Exercise:

Breathe in, lengthen your spine, and exhale, hinge at your hips to reach forward.

Hold onto your shins, ankles, or feet.

Inhale to elongate, and exhale to deepen the stretch, feeling the release in your lower back and hamstrings.

Knee Hugs

Starting Position:

Stand with feet hip-width apart.

Exercise:

Get one knee lifted towards your chest, holding it with both hands.

Hug the knee gently, feeling a stretch in your hip flexor.

Switch to the other leg, alternating in a rhythmic motion.

Side-to-Side Head Tilts

Starting Position:

Sit or stand with a straight spine.

Exercise:

Inhale, tilt your head to one side, bringing your ear towards your shoulder.

Exhale, return to the centre and tilt to the other side.

Repeat, feeling a gentle stretch along the side of your neck.

Dynamic Arm Swings

Starting Position:

Stand with feet shoulder-width apart.

Exercise:

Swing your arms forward and backward in a controlled manner.

Gradually increase the range of motion, incorporating the entire shoulder joint.

Focus on the fluidity of the movement.

Lumbar Rotation

Starting Position:

Sit on the floor with legs crossed.

Exercise:

Breath in, lengthen your spine.

Exhale, twist your torso to one side, placing one hand behind you and the other on your knee.

Inhale back to the center and repeat on the other side.

Engage your core and feel the gentle stretch in your lower back.

Calf Raises

Starting Position:

Stand with feet hip-width apart.

Exercise:

Inhale, lift your heels off the ground, rising onto your toes.

Exhale, lower your heels back down.

Repeat, feeling the stretch and activation in your calf muscles.

Thoracic Spine Extension

Starting Position:

Kneel on all fours with hands under shoulders.

Exercise:

Inhale, arch your back, lifting your chest towards the ceiling.

Exhale, round your spine.

Repeat, focusing on mobilizing your upper back.

Seated Side Stretch

Starting Position:

Sit cross-legged.

Exercise:

Breath in, lengthen your spine.

Exhale, lean to one side, bringing your hand towards the floor.

Inhale back to the centre and repeat on the other side.

Feel the stretch along your side and through your waist.

Quad Stretch

Starting Position:

Stand with feet hip-width apart.

Exercise:

Lift one foot towards your glutes, holding the ankle with your hand.

Feel the stretch in your quadriceps.

Switch to the other leg, alternating in a controlled manner.

Seated Twist

Starting Position:

Sit with legs extended in front of you.

Exercise:

Inhale, lengthen your spine.

Exhale, twist your torso to one side, placing one hand behind you and the other on your knee.

Inhale back to the centre and repeat on the other side.

Engage your core and enjoy the spinal rotation.

Desk Exercises for Office Workers

Seated Spinal Twist

Starting Position:

Get seated comfortably in your chair with a straight spine.

Exercise:

Breath in, lengthen your spine.

Exhale, twist your torso to one side, placing one hand on the opposite knee and the other on the back of your chair.

Inhale back to the centre and repeat on the other side.

Engage your core and feel the gentle stretch in your spine.

Desk Chair Squats

Starting Position:

Stand in front of your desk with feet hip-width apart.

Exercise:

Breath out, sit back into a squat position like you were going to sit in your chair.

Exhale, push through your heels to stand back up.

Repeat for the duration, engaging your glutes and thighs.

Maintain good posture throughout the movement.

Chair Leg Lifts

Starting Position:

Get seated on the edge of your chair with a straight back.

Exercise:

Get one leg lifted straight out in front of you, engaging your core.

Hold for a while and lower the leg.

Repeat on the other leg.

Focus on controlled movements, feeling the activation in your abdominal muscles.

Wrist and Forearm Stretch

Starting Position:

Get your arm extended in front of you, palm facing down.

Exercise:

Use your opposite hand to gently pull back on your fingers, stretching the wrist and forearm.

Hold for a few breaths, then switch to the other hand.

Perform this stretch to relieve tension from typing and mouse use.

Seated Knee Tucks

Starting Position:

Sit on the edge of your chair with knees bent and feet flat on the floor.

Exercise:

Inhale, lift one knee towards your chest, hugging it with both hands.

Exhale, lower the foot back to the floor.

Switch to the other leg, alternating in a controlled manner.

Engage your core and feel the activation in your lower abdominal muscles.

Desk Chair Twists

Starting Position:

Sit in your chair with a straight spine.

Exercise:

Breath in, reach one arm across your body and place it on the opposite armrest or back of the chair.

Exhale, twist your torso gently, looking over your shoulder.

Inhale back to the centre and repeat on the other side.

Feel the stretch along your spine and through your obliques.

Seated Shoulder Opener

Starting Position:

Sit comfortably, bringing your hands behind your back, fingers interlaced.

Exercise:

Inhale, straighten your arms, and lift them slightly.

Exhale, opening your chest and squeezing your shoulder blades together.

Inhale, release the stretch slightly, and exhale to deepen.

Feel the stretch across your chest and shoulders.

Desk Hamstring Stretch

Starting Position:

Sit on the edge of your chair with one leg extended straight and the other foot flat on the floor.

Exercise:

Inhale, lengthen your spine.

Breath out, hinge at your hips, reaching towards your toes.

Inhale back to the center, feeling the stretch in your hamstrings.

Switch to the other leg and repeat.

Calf Raises at Your Desk

Starting Position:

Sit in your chair with both feet flat on the floor.

Exercise:

Inhale, lift your heels off the ground, rising onto the balls of your feet.

Exhale, lower your heels back down.

Repeat, feeling the activation in your calf muscles.

This exercise helps improve circulation and lower leg strength.

Seated Figure-Four Stretch

Starting Position:

Sit tall in your chair with both feet flat on the floor.

Exercise:

Lift one foot and place the ankle on the opposite knee, creating a figure-four shape.

Inhale, sit up straight, and exhale, gently press on the lifted knee to deepen the stretch.

Hold for a few breaths, feeling the stretch in your hip.

Switch to the other leg and repeat.

Bonus: Somatic Diet Recipes

Breakfast Recipes

1. Berry and Yogurt Parfait

Ingredients:

1 cup of low-fat Greek yogurt

Half cup of mixed berries (strawberries, blueberries, raspberries)

2 tablespoons of honey

1/4 cup of granola

Instructions:

In a glass, layer Greek yogurt, mixed berries, and honey or a bowl.

Sprinkle granola on top.

Enjoy this nutritious and satisfying parfait.

2. Avocado and Spinach Breakfast Wrap

Ingredients:

1 whole-grain tortilla

1/2 ripe avocado, sliced

Handful of fresh spinach leaves

2 eggs, scrambled

Salt and pepper to taste

Instructions:

Place the whole-grain tortilla on a clean surface.

Layer avocado slices, fresh spinach leaves, and scrambled eggs.

Season with salt and pepper.

Roll up the tortilla and enjoy a protein-packed breakfast wrap.

3. Oatmeal with Almonds and Banana

Ingredients:

1/2 cup of rolled oats

1 cup of almond milk

1 banana, sliced

Handful of chopped almonds

1 teaspoon of honey (optional)

Instructions:

Cook rolled oats with almond milk according to package instructions.

Top with banana slices and chopped almonds.

Drizzle honey if desired.

A hearty and filling breakfast is ready.

Lunch Recipes

4. Quinoa and Chickpea Salad

Ingredients:

1 cup of cooked quinoa

1 cup of chickpeas, drained and rinsed

1 cucumber, diced

1 red bell pepper, chopped

Handful of fresh parsley, chopped

Juice of 1 lemon

Olive oil, salt, and pepper to taste

Instructions:

In a large bowl, combine cooked quinoa, chickpeas, cucumber, red bell pepper, and fresh parsley.

Drizzle using the lemon juice and olive oil, and season with salt and pepper.

Toss well and enjoy this refreshing and nutritious salad.

5. Grilled Chicken and Vegetable Wrap

Ingredients:

4 oz grilled chicken breast, sliced

1 whole-grain wrap

1/2 cup mixed grilled vegetables (zucchini, bell peppers, onions)

2 tablespoons of hummus

Fresh spinach leaves

Instructions:

Lay the whole-grain wrap on a clean surface.

Spread hummus on the wrap.

Add sliced grilled chicken, grilled vegetables, and fresh spinach.

Roll up the wrap and enjoy a protein-rich lunch.

Dinner Recipes

6. Baked Salmon with Asparagus

Ingredients:

6 oz salmon fillet

1 bunch of asparagus

1 lemon, sliced

1 tablespoon of olive oil

Salt, pepper, and dill to taste

Instructions:

Preheat the oven to 375°F (190°C).

On a baking sheet, place salmon and asparagus.

Drizzle with olive oil, season with salt, pepper, and dill.

Add lemon slices on top.

Bake for 20-25 minutes until salmon is cooked through and asparagus is tender.

7. Lentil and Vegetable Stir-Fry

Ingredients:

One cup of cooked green or brown lentils

1 cup of mixed stir-fry vegetables (bell peppers, broccoli, snap peas)

1/4 cup of low-sodium soy sauce

1 tablespoon of sesame oil

2 cloves of garlic, minced

1 teaspoon of ginger, grated

Instructions:

Heat sesame oil over moderate heat in a large pan.

Include the minced garlic and grated ginger, and sauté for two minutes.

Add mixed vegetables and cooked lentils, stir-fry for 5-7 minutes.

Pour soy sauce over the mixture and cook for an additional 2 minutes.

Smoothie Recipe

8. Green Protein Smoothie

Ingredients:

1 cup of spinach leaves

1/2 banana

1/2 cup of Greek yogurt

1 tablespoon of almond butter

1 cup of almond milk

Ice cubes (optional)

Instructions:

Blend spinach, banana, Greek yogurt, almond butter, and almond milk until smooth.

Add ice cubes if desired for a colder consistency.

Enjoy a protein-packed green smoothie to kickstart your day.

Juice Recipes

9. Citrus and Carrot Juice

Ingredients:

2 oranges, peeled and segmented

2 carrots, washed and chopped

1 lemon, peeled and sliced

1-inch piece of ginger

1/2 cup of water

Instructions:

Place oranges, carrots, lemon, ginger, and water in a juicer.

Process until you get a fresh and vibrant citrus and carrot juice.

10. Green Detox Juice

Ingredients:

1 cucumber, peeled and sliced

2 celery stalks

Handful of kale leaves

1 green apple, cored and sliced

1/2 lemon, peeled

Instructions:

Put cucumber, celery, kale, green apple, and lemon through a juicer.

Pour the green detox juice into a glass and enjoy the cleansing flavors.

SECTION III

Integrating Somatic Exercises into Your Routine

In this section, we provide tools to help you build a consistent somatic exercise routine into your daily life. Establishing regular somatic practice is key to experiencing the full benefits to body, mind and spirit.

We will outline a structured 4 week somatic workout plan you can follow, day-by-day. This removes the guesswork of what exercises to do each day.

Each day has two morning and two evening routines outlined, drawing from these somatic exercise categories.

In addition, we provide a journal template to record your experiences with each exercise session. Writing about your practice helps instill it as a habit and track your progress. Noticing improvements in how you feel gives motivational feedback.

Finally, we include a somatic exercise tracker chart you can use to check off each completed routine. This helps build accountability and consistency week-to-week in your practice. You can note any modifications or reflections after each session.

Our goal is to simplify starting and sticking with a regular somatic exercise routine. By following the structured 4 week plan, using the journal to record your journey, and checking off sessions in your tracker, you build sustainable somatic habits. In a month's time, you are likely to feel dramatic mind-body benefits that inspire you to continue the practices long-term

4 Weeks Workout Plan

Week 1

Day 1:

Morning: Pelvic Tilts (Core Activation - Exercise 1)

Evening: Neck and Shoulder Rolls (Mobility - Exercise 1)

Day 2:

Morning: Seated Russian Twists (Core Activation - Exercise 4)

Evening: Spinal Flexibility Movements (Mobility - Exercise 2)

Day 3:

Morning: Plank with Hip Dips (Core Activation - Exercise 7)

Evening: Hip Circles (Mobility - Exercise 3)

Day 4:

Morning: Leg Raises (Core Activation - Exercise 8)

Evening: Ankle Rolls (Mobility - Exercise 4)

Day 5:

Morning: Standing Side Bend (Core Activation - Exercise 12)

Evening: Wrist and Hand Stretches (Mobility - Exercise 5)

Day 6:

Morning: Bicycle Crunches (Core Activation - Exercise 6)

Evening: Seated Forward Bend (Mobility - Exercise 6)

Day 7:

Morning: Side Plank (Core Activation - Exercise 9)

Evening: Knee Hugs (Mobility - Exercise 7)

Week 2

Day 8:

Morning: Rolling Like a Ball (Core Activation - Exercise 11)

Evening: Dynamic Arm Swings (Mobility - Exercise 9)

Day 9:

Morning: Reverse Crunches (Core Activation - Exercise 14)

Evening: Lumbar Rotation (Mobility - Exercise 10)

Day 10:

Morning: Standing Knee-to-Elbow Crunch (Core Activation - Exercise 15)

Evening: Calf Raises at Your Desk (Mobility - Exercise 11)

Day 11:

Morning: Seated Figure-Four Stretch (Mobility - Exercise 10)

Evening: Desk Chair Squats (Core Activation - Exercise 2)

Day 12:

Morning: Cat-Cow Stretch (Core Activation - Exercise 5)

Evening: Seated Knee Tucks (Core Activation - Exercise 5)

Day 13:

Morning: Twisting Waist Movements (Core Activation - Exercise 3)

Evening: Thoracic Spine Extension (Mobility - Exercise 12)

Day 14:

Morning: Hollow Body Hold (Core Activation - Exercise 10)

Evening: Quad Stretch (Mobility - Exercise 14)

Week 3

Day 15:

Morning: Desk Chair Twists (Mobility - Exercise 6)

Evening: Seated Shoulder Opener (Mobility - Exercise 7)

Day 16:

Morning: Seated Neck Tilts (Mobility - Exercise 8)

Evening: Chair Leg Lifts (Core Activation - Exercise 3)

Day 17:

Morning: Spinal Flexibility Movements (Mobility - Exercise 2)

Evening: Dynamic Arm Swings (Mobility - Exercise 9)

Day 18:

Morning: Desk Hamstring Stretch (Mobility - Exercise 8)

Evening: Reverse Crunches (Core Activation - Exercise 14)

Day 19:

Morning: Seated Forward Bend (Mobility - Exercise 6)

Evening: Wrist and Forearm Stretch (Mobility - Exercise 5)

Day 20:

Morning: Side Plank (Core Activation - Exercise 9)

Evening: Seated Figure-Four Stretch (Mobility - Exercise 10)

Day 21:

Morning: Cat-Cow Stretch (Core Activation - Exercise 5)

Evening: Standing Side Bend (Core Activation - Exercise 12)

Week 4

Day 22:

Morning: Rolling Like a Ball (Core Activation - Exercise 11)

Evening: Seated Neck Tilts (Mobility - Exercise 8)

Day 23:

Morning: Standing Knee-to-Elbow Crunch (Core Activation - Exercise 15)

Evening: Dynamic Arm Swings (Mobility - Exercise 9)

Day 24:

Morning: Reverse Crunches (Core Activation - Exercise 14)

Evening: Desk Chair Squats (Core Activation - Exercise 2)

Day 25:

Morning: Seated Knee Tucks (Core Activation - Exercise 5)

Evening: Seated Figure-Four Stretch (Mobility - Exercise 10)

Day 26:

Morning: Hollow Body Hold (Core Activation - Exercise 10)

Evening: Quad Stretch (Mobility - Exercise 14)

Day 27:

Morning: Cat-Cow Stretch (Core Activation - Exercise 5)

Evening: Seated Hamstring Stretch (Mobility - Exercise 6)

Day 28:

Morning: Twisting Waist Movements (Core Activation - Exercise 3)

Evening: Wrist and Forearm Stretch (Mobility - Exercise 5)

Journal and Tracker User Guide

Welcome to the Somatic Exercise Journal and Tracker, your dedicated space to record and reflect on your 4-week somatic movement journey. This journal will support you in building mind-body awareness and sticking with regular somatic practice.

Journal Structure

The somatic exercise journal is structured into 4 weekly workout trackers, with space each day to log your morning and evening practices. You can note the specific exercises, duration, and any helpful reflections. Tick each box as you complete sessions to see your progress stacking up.

After each week is a reflection note page. Here you can write about your experiences that week – challenges, benefits noticed, insights gained, positive changes emerging. Notice patterns over the month.

Additional tracker templates and reflection pages are provided to continue your somatic exercise routine beyond the 4 weeks if you desire. This journal can evolve with you.

Using the Journal

When using your somatic exercise journal:

- Record exercises done each day, even quick informal practices. Every mindful moment counts.

- Note details like duration, reps, modifications, intensity. Observe how these change.

- Reflect on sensations, breath, focus level. What did you learn about your body and mind?

- Tick each box with satisfaction as you persist through the 4 weeks. Let it be a visual mark of your dedication.

- In reflection pages, describe your inner experiences. Appreciate growth and insights gained.

- Re-read previous weeks to see your progression. Celebrate successes and growth.

This somatic journal is more than a log of exercises done. It is a space to deepen your inner awareness and relationship with your whole self – body, mind, spirit. Let it guide you in integrating the principles of somatics into your daily living.

Conclusion

The journey into somatic movement starts with a single mindful step - a commitment to reconnecting with your body's inner wisdom. Through the gentle practices of somatic exercises, you learn to undo habitual tension, quiet your thinking mind, and tune into subtle physical sensations. Rather than forcing progress, you move with compassionate awareness.

An anti-inflammatory, whole foods diet provides nourishment to support your mind-body exploration. Conscious breathing techniques empower you to manage stress and access deeper states of calm.

Developing somatic competency is a process of unlearning – shedding patterns of exertion and disconnect. With patience and daily practice, you come home to yourself. Pain and anxiety yield to presence.

This book has outlined foundations and tools to guide you in awakening to the possibilities of the somatic path. Our hope is that the knowledge gained inspires you to continue your embodied evolution.

While the exercises herein are simple, their effects are profound. Movement becomes meditation when infused with mindful attention. You repattern the nervous system, resolve trauma in the tissues, and integrate all aspects of your being.

Trust in the innate inner wisdom of your body. Lean into sensorial experience. Let somatic exercises help you feel more at home, peaceful and empowered in your skin. Keep exploring this catalytic realm of healing connection.

The somatic journey is nothing short of a remembrance of your wholeness. May this book begin an expansive process of coming home to You.

BONUS: TRACKER AND JOURNAL

SOMATIC EXERCISE TRACKER		
DAYS	**EXERCISES**	**MARK**

REFLECTION NOTE

REFLECTION NOTE

REFLECTION NOTE

REFLECTION NOTE

SOMATIC EXERCISE TRACKER

DAYS	EXERCISES	MARK

REFLECTION NOTE

REFLECTION NOTE

REFLECTION NOTE

SOMATIC EXERCISE TRACKER

DAYS	EXERCISES	MARK

REFLECTION NOTE

REFLECTION NOTE

REFLECTION NOTE

REFLECTION NOTE

SOMATIC EXERCISE TRACKER

DAYS	EXERCISES	MARK

REFLECTION NOTE

REFLECTION NOTE

REFLECTION NOTE

REFLECTION NOTE

REFLECTION NOTE

REFLECTION NOTE

REFLECTION NOTE

REFLECTION NOTE

REFLECTION NOTE

REFLECTION NOTE

REFLECTION NOTE